BENDING THE CURVE

An American Healthcare Imperative

by

R.W. Murphy

MBA, REBC, ChFC, RHU, CLU

Aqua Clara Press
Clearwater, FL
June 2019

R.W. Murphy

This Page Left Blank

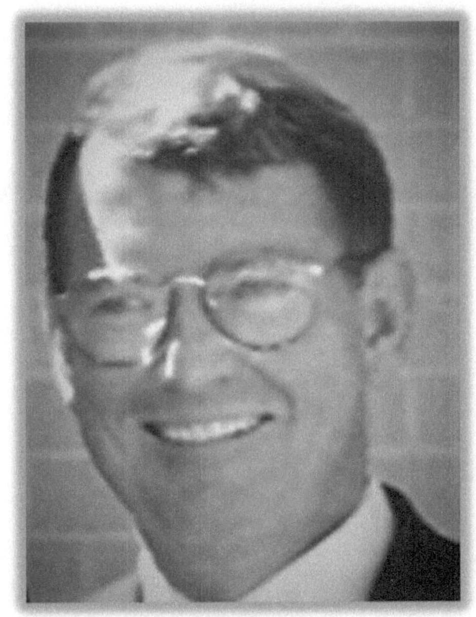

Author

R.W. Murphy

R.W. Murphy

INTRODUCTION

written by
Carlos F.X. Rodriguez, FACHE
Senior Healthcare Administrator
West Palm Beach, Florida

First, let me acknowledge that Carlos F.X. Rodriguez is a pseudonym. I am not sure how much pushback this book will receive in the in healthcare industry. Because the welfare of my family is dependent on my career as a professional administrator, I can't afford to be a lightning rod. Nevertheless, I felt that it was important to make a few candid comments about "Bending the Curve: An American Healthcare Imperative." Writing the Introduction under an alias has allowed me to do so.

The book is short but it is also very much on point. R.W. Murphy has indeed been in the trenches since healthcare became a problem for employers in the early 1980s. However, he leaves out a part of his curriculum vitae. In 1985 he was offered a position working for a for-profit hospital company in Southern California. He came very close to coming over to the dark side. Indeed, according to his version of events, had it not been for the fact that an insurance company that was simultaneously bidding for his services sent a moving van to his home and absconded with all his personal effects, he might have ended up on my side of many of these issues.

I met him in 1995. He had been retained to build an "anti-managed care" insurance product by a person who is known as an icon in medical education. The physician community was still very angry about the impositions MCOs were forcing on their lives. As a result, his client was willing to spend a lot of personal money to counter the trend. In essence, Murphy planned to take all the good things he had learned from fifteen years of costs control initiatives and toss out all the bad ones. He intended to reimburse physician claims on a schedule as a percentage of Medicare. He had an actuary in Princeton, NJ evaluate the plan design and lined up an insurance company to stand behind it. He also had an administrative interface set up with a firm in Philadelphia, PA. The initial product offering was to be in Florida and he had legal opinions rendered to ensure it didn't run afoul of regulators. A Dallas-based attorney who was an expert on ERISA law was retained to weigh in on related issues. Lastly, Murphy started initial negotiations to set up a risk-bearing reinsurance company in the Caribbean. It was actually an elegant plan. The problem was that it was ten or more years before its time.

Once again, with this book he is looking out into the future with unusually discerning eyes. Some of his suggestions might appear to be premature. Yet, it's hard to dispute his underlying thesis about costs and demand. One might dispute his conclusions about inevitability and the alternative ways to prevent a cataclysm. In fact, people in the healthcare industry will likely dispute his description of present and past dynamics.

Nonetheless, one thing can't be challenged – the importance of Americans to be sensitive to all the arguments he puts forth as a key election approaches. Even if they reject them, at least the concepts will have been considered. An equally important corollary he proffers is that Americans must be prepared to make educated choices and not react simply to the rhetoric of demagogues with vested interests. Related to all that is his suggestion to the public that it not be cowed by what he calls "hot words." He encourages people to learn the true nature of suggested alternative policies and reject rhetoric designed to appeal to fear. He implicitly indicates that Americans cede their franchise as the ultimate source of governance if they fail to do so.

He calls it "an American healthcare imperative" and indicates that is existential to the US over the relatively near-term. He doesn't specify; however, I take that to mean twenty to fifty years into the future. He argues emphatically, that something as large and complex as the US healthcare delivery system must start its turn now to head off disaster by then. I have heard him refer to it as turning an aircraft carrier – not a speedboat.

Coming primarily from the hospital business - and being pretty right-leaning politically – I can't give R.W. Murphy's analysis a blanket blessing. However, I unequivocally give him credit for being the soothsayer that I have always known him to be. The paradigm likely won't be shifted precisely as he describes it. However, the fact that it is shifted at all will be due to people like him. Those who have similar scholarly honesty and face the challenges of innovation bravely will be the healthcare leaders of the future.

CFXR

Table of Contents

PROLOGUE: *STEALING MY OWN THUNDER*

What is the curve to which I refer in the title you might ask. Secondly, you might want to know why I call it an American healthcare imperative. The answers to both questions are actually not complex. However, execution of solutions is quite another matter.

However, before going on, I want to inject a question of my own. Why do economists and statisticians insist on calling straight lines "curves?" I'll talk a lot about a rigid demand curve. Although in reality, it is as straight as a freshly sawn piece of white oak at an Alabama sawmill.

There lies the rub. The US healthcare delivery system is virtually perfectly inelastic. For those without economics degrees, let it suffice to say that we will purchase the same amount of healthcare services no matter what price we are charged for them. In fact, we will actually purchase incrementally more over time due to practice dynamics. Sadly, no matter how much financial pain is induced individually, the aggregate market behavior doesn't change. In many ways we are actually healthcare junkies.

Yet, it is a totally unsustainable model over time. The unit cost of services in the US is far higher than any other developed country in the world. That is an indictment in and by itself. However, the real danger lies in the fact that there is no structural change on the horizon whereby our systemic cost acceleration will be abated. Small nips at utilization control and broader risk pools are nothing more than window dressing relative to the real problem.

I consider myself more left leaning than right when it comes to healthcare. However, I concur with the GOP on one issue: ACA was never the answer to runaway costs. At best, it was the most recent stair step measure. The acceleration in per capita claims and premiums was reduced by adding mandated "young healthies" into the system (*i.e.,* those who will pay premiums but not incur substantial claims). However, the new baseline was just the foundation for the same percentage growth in costs we have witnessed for decades – perhaps more. Any professional healthcare economist who says they didn't see it coming needs to go back to their alma mater for some retraining. It was intuitively obvious from the start to the most casual observer. The only way insurance carriers were going to keep premiums down was annual reduction in benefits. That was exacerbated by foolish pricing structures that assumed more market share than ever occurred. So, they were underpriced on day one; didn't get the incremental healthy risk pool growth they anticipated; and, were still subject to all the cost drivers that existed pre-ACA. It was like General Custer was driving the ship [please excuse the mixed metaphor]. The truth is that the first two elements can be addressed relatively easily by national healthcare policy decisions. Pricing can be made right and the risk pools can be enhanced. I said "relatively" because I recognize the political third rail "mandating" has become. Moreover, the influence of the incremental enrollment – while positive – is marginal. The actual elephant in the room is that damn inelasticity thing.

I reject out of hand the notion that patient behavior will ever change enough to impact the underlying cost structure. I was personally involved with all types of attempts at utilization management in the '80s and '90s – from benefit-dependent second opinions to heavy handed HMO medical directors. They took a couple of basis points off an employer's annual healthcare bill (*n.b.*, and that of the feds too); however, they didn't slow down the percentage growth in the underlying cost structure an iota.

The US in the last few years has been drifting away from a true laissez-faire wholesale market for healthcare component products. Implied threats to the developers and manufacturers by politicians have depressed unit pricing acceleration a tad. Nonetheless, it would be the height of naivety to believe the same forces are not just temporarily lurking in the shadows waiting for a more pliable administration. When they re-emerge, it will be with a vengeance; they will do all they can to recover lost revenues from the lean years. The elasticity curve will once again be as straight as that Alabama board.

The question is not whether it should be bent. There is a clear existential argument that says it must. The question is actually how to accomplish that. I only see three possible ways. Actually it might only be two due to one being clothed as another.

The first is via the governmental regulation route. Ultimately, there needs to be downward pressure applied to the sources of healthcare goods and services [read here a substantial bending of the elasticity curve]. Simultaneously, the tendency of every small town to want the Taj Mahal of hospitals in their community needs to be dampened. Hypothetically, both could be accomplished through legislation. Pragmatically, that's merely a pipe dream. Indeed, one large southern state just enacted legislation that will allow hospital sprawl statewide – actual need notwithstanding.

The other route might be a single-payer system whereby the federal government takes on all the financial risk. It could choose whatever level of payment for services it thought fair – essentially forcing the curve to be bent. Since the "US One Plan" (my imaginary name for it) would be the only game in town, the producers who had sucked on the hind teet of inelasticity since the late 70s would no longer be able to set prices arbitrarily. Of course, they would also scream that US One Plan damaged the integrity of the entire healthcare delivery system; they would immediately point to the state-of-the-art innovation that their pricing has historically allowed by funding research and development. That's actually a banal, well-worn mantra of Big Pharma. Moreover, there are several things to which they won't point such as the Porsches all lined up in the parking lot; the multi-million dollar bonuses paid to officers; the upward slope of their common stock valuation over time; the average level of pay in the industry in general; and the tiny windows of time over which goodwill is amortized for new product rollouts. Of those, the last might be the most despicable.

Whereas the payback period for a new item could easily be twenty years, it might indeed only be planned at five. Of that, the US market pays an inordinate share of the incremental expense that is passed along (*e.g.*, a million dollars in R&D investment on a twenty year goodwill schedule might allow $50,000 per year to be expensed; a five year schedule would allow $200,000 for the exact same item). It also causes a skewed positive impact on earnings in the sixth year. I don't suggest here that investment in research should be curtailed. I do suggest that amortization should be flattened and that domestic and foreign pricing be more balanced. Joe Lunchbucket, his family and his employer should not be financing the welfare of a manufacturer via crushing premiums and point of service cost sharing; especially when someone on the other side of the world is utilizing the same product for 10-20% of the US cost.

I actually see a third way the curve might be bent. However, it might require anti-trust regulation to be waived. What if blocks of insurance companies formed purchasing pools? Instead of the US One Plan making all the purchasing decisions via the federal government, maybe there could be three divisions - East, Central and West. Perhaps setting up three specialty logistics companies – totally arms-length from insurance marketing and underwriting results – would be the way to go. Once again, they would have to have the authority to contract with providers of goods and services anywhere in the world. They should publically state their mission – *i.e.*, to solely bend the curve. The three divisions might also be owned by a central holding company to insure uniformity and inter-divisional cooperation. Without getting too far afield in my thinking here, perhaps a Federal

Reserve type structure might work with the holding company's board being akin to the Board of Governors. You might ask why I suggest the involvement of the insurance companies. The answer is twofold; they have gained significant experience in wholesale contacting over the managed care years; and, participation would keep them from feeling like they had been disenfranchised by the new model.

Ultimately, it seems to me that either the US One Plan or the regional divisions system could allow all comers to participate at Medicare level costs or - if the curve is substantially bent- perhaps even below. If the regional divisions model was adopted, I could foresee a risk-sharing arrangement between the insurance companies and the US government. On the front-end it would look to the average citizen like not much had changed – a policy would be issued on company paper; on the back-end it would be drastically different. In some ways it would compare to the way Medicare uses insurance companies as their administrative interface from region to region. Although, in this case I would suggest that the insurance companies continue to have downside financial risk – essentially a little skin in the game.

Politicians and healthcare gurus can scream forever about pre-existing exclusions and heavy handed mandates. However, note that not a single viable alternative to ACA has emerged after two years of the current administration's dominance and a receptive Senate. It's not because they don't want to repeal and replace ACA. The fact is they don't know how. Indeed, they can't even define what it is they are shooting at beyond raising the specter of the last administration. As you will see in the following section, that is actually quite a common problem. The perception of what constitutes "healthcare reform" varies from interest group to interest group.

I don't want to give the left a free pass on all these issues. Most of the initiatives to date coming from that side are poorly founded. Ultimately, they might make sense; however, not a single candidate can say in fine detail how they would get from where we are today to where they suggest we should be. Two examples of inept execution come to mind: the Medicaid Christmas tree and the IRS/HHS regulatory storm associated with ACA. The actual events were wholly unexpected by the most ardent supporters of each.

✳✳✳

As I said above, bending the curve is actually an existential imperative. It is not just for the viability of the healthcare delivery system. The financial consequences are actually devastating on both micro and macro levels. What happens when limited family resources have to be allocated between healthcare and college for the kids? Sooner or later US society will inevitably be dumbed down in the aggregate. On the macro level one must accept the fact that there are only a finite number of dollars in the US economy – the Fed adding to the money supply notwithstanding. If healthcare expenditures are rising as a percent of GDP, what is being foregone in the process? Indeed, what has already been foregone relative to what might have been?

The manufacturers would argue that the incremental dollars are being reinvested in the health of society and therefore have substantial investment value. I can remember the graduate professor of finance I had while working on my MBA. He would have us rank every alternative investment by net present value and internal rate of return. I'm not sure I could even define the actual investment in healthcare dollars. Where did the incremental money actually get spent and on what? I certainly couldn't compute a net present value for the alleged investment. Yet, I could easily do so for a dozen infrastructure investments around the US. Crumbling bridges are obvious; less so are Big Pharma shots at blockbuster drugs that turn out to be duds.

* * *

I will reach back to my Irish roots for hyperbole here. We must bend the curve or perish. Less dramatically said – ignoring it isn't an option any longer. Those white haired men in DC might last it out; however, their grandchildren certainly won't. I have couched all my above comments in economic imperative terms. Let me adjust that a bit. It's also a moral imperative. I'm not talking about the morality associated with 28 million Americans not having formalized healthcare. In fact, I mean the fiduciary obligation US leaders have to all Americans. To that end, I would prefer the show-boaters stand aside and let the professionals go to work.

– R.W. Murphy

CHAPTER I: *WHAT IS THE ISSUE*

In 1980, I had no idea I was being recruited for war. However, indeed I was – the First Healthcare War had just begun. As an ex-naval officer, I thought I had seen my last of that kind of thing. What I didn't know was that it was to be a new kind of war. It might even be considered a civil war of sorts since no engagements were ever fought outside US territory. Thirty nine years later, the war still persists. The fronts have shifted slightly since '80. However, it has been like intractable trench warfare; there has never been any kind of decisive victory. I can point to two major campaigns and half a dozen skirmishes. Yet, no substantial terrain has been gained nor has the *casus belli* been assuaged meaningfully.

Quite incongruously, the *casus belli* per se remains illusory for many. In 2004 I was a participant for six days at a course called Skills for the New World of Healthcare. It was conducted jointly by:

- Harvard Medical School
- Harvard School of Public Health
- Harvard JFK School of Government
- Harvard Div. of Health Policy Research & Education

There were forty participants from all over the US. It had been advertised as an eclectic grouping of professionals with concerns about healthcare policy. As a consultant, I thought the course might be valuable to me professionally. However, the Harvard folks had left a few key pieces of info out of their web blurb. It was originally sponsored by the Academy of Thoracic Surgeons. Of the forty participants, thirty were surgeons – mostly cardiac specialists. I never pressed for details; however, it seemed that virtually all of them were on some form of scholarship as the best and brightest from their respective communities. Five other participants were administrators or board members from hospitals. There were three foreign participants. There was also an aide to a US congressman.

Lastly, there was me. As a side note, I should mention that only one participant was a woman - one of the hospital administrators.

On the second day of classroom work, I was convinced that I had made a dreadful error. The gray matter massed in the room was awe inspiring; indeed, it made me feel like a pretender. I had already checked schedules from Boston's North Station and Logan Airport when I approached the retired, thoracic surgeon who was the course's ad hoc director. The train schedule check was due to a stop I had to make with relatives who lived fifteen miles north of Boston before leaving town. I told the director that I was certain that I had made a mistake enrolling; I was going to bail and eat the associated costs – roughly $5,000 tuition plus expenses (*n.b.*, about $6,800 in 2019).

He pulled me aside and chatted with me as a doc might chat with a sick patient. He explained to me that my presence there was not a mistake. In fact, it was quite a deliberate decision on the part of the faculty. Yes, the people in the room were incredibly gifted. However, they existed in a rarified atmosphere. He indicated that someone like me was required for gravitas – essentially a real world anchor. Somehow, he knew that I had been fighting the war for twenty-four years. Conversely, some of the cardiac specialists were barely thirty-five years old. The bottom line: he convinced me to not quit. I was never so glad that I did as he suggested. It was the second time in my life I thought I was outclassed only to find that we each have our own relative strengths.

So why do I mention all of that? Of forty participants, when asked to each list the ten things broken with the US healthcare delivery system in priority order, not one list was the same, albeit the top five issues came up repeatedly in random order. Related to that was another lack of consistency. The forty participants were placed in six workgroups to address one specific broken item each and report out to the faculty. A presentation was to be made the afternoon of the last day. My group selected the issue of how to provide medical care to the segment of the population that makes too much money to participate in Medicaid but can't afford monthly premiums and point of service costs (*i.e.*, multiple deductibles, copays and coinsurance, etc.).

From Monday to Wednesday, members of my workgroup fought every night without even getting close to compromise. Moreover, it was on our own personal time; we gathered to work on the project each night after a late dinner and speaker in the JFK School penthouse. As a general rule, driven people don't like to fail; as such, none of my colleagues wanted to deliver a half-baked product to the faculty on Friday. It ended up that Thursday became compromise day. The barriers came down and an excellent presentation was developed. Unfortunately, I was the one selected to stand in the well and deliver it the next day.

My point: at times, the brightest medical professionals in the world cannot agree on the issues or the fixes. When you hear the phrase "healthcare reform," what actually is it that is being fixed? Most American's cannot answer that question. It is my opinion that they are used like pawns by politicians who claim to have absolute prescience on such.

CHAPTER II: *SUPPLY AND DEMAND*

The vast majority of Americans consider the healthcare problem to be a financial one. Their perception is based on how much is deducted from their paycheck each week to participate in an employee-sponsored health plan as well as its related point of service costs. Due to various factors, in the last fifteen years employees have seen an unprecedented acceleration in the costs they bear. To them, runaway employee cost is the issue.

Employers find themselves in the same frame of mind. Healthcare was once a perk for their employees. It has since become a burden. An employer now often has to announce the bad news annually. Premiums and cost-sharing go up for employees and benefit levels come down – at the fastest level in the last forty years. At some point, many plans become so financially unwieldy that employers are forced to terminate them. To them, insurance companies and high premiums are the problems.

Before the advent of the ACA in 2010, the number of those uninsured in the US was estimated to be 40 million. If you accept that the number of working age adults in the US is 243 million that equates to roughly 16.5% of adult Americans. The most recent figure pegs it at 28 million uninsured or about 11.5%. Regardless of the accuracy, it's a huge number under any circumstances. Social scientists point to the impact of having a relatively sicker population than other countries. Hospitals and providers point to cost shifting. Some people do indeed die due to lack of formalized medical coverage; however the fact is that most don't – some entity picks up the tab for a modicum of care.

Others will point to the US having an unconscionable morbidity rate – especially in certain segments of its population - relative to all other developed nations worldwide. Infant mortality is an oft-cited statistic in that argument.

Some younger observers will indicate that the biggest problem is that an undue amount of resources is devoted to people at the very end of their lives. Related to that argument, they will indicate that fee-for-service Medicare utilization is regularly abused by both patients and providers. Indeed, I believe both to be true.

Older patients often get tests with very little marginal efficacy since the last time they were run – often annually when a five year cycle would be clinically sound practice. However, overutilization is a matter of perception; its importance is questionable in the big scheme of things.

Of course, any consideration of restricting provider services must address tort reform. Providers are quick to indicate that the only reason they give so many tests is that they are afraid of being sued. In the case of Medicare patients, there are two related factors: how family members perceive their loved one's treatment regimen (*i.e.* will the family sue); and, what kind of geriatric, comparative network exists (*i.e.*, what did a friend get from their doc for the same thing). In the fee-for-service Medicare sector, a waste factor of 20% is estimated by many – time of life considerations notwithstanding.

SUPPLY SIDE COST ACCELERATION

Ultimately, the biggest issue is cost. Virtually all the other issues above are interrelated and downstream from that. Cost creep has been an issue in the US healthcare delivery system since third parties began paying the majority of the aggregate US healthcare bill. In the insurance industry the term is "annual trend." It is not simply inflation; it also reflects structural and dynamic changes in the system from year to year. It's a going-forward projection so it's always no more than a best bet figure. Sometimes, the actuaries are not dead on; however, rarely do they miss by much.

In recent years cost creep has become systemically untenable. The slope of the curve has become more acute at a time when the percentage of household income for medical care has grown to the breaking point for many. Bottom line: the rate of increase in costs is accelerating at a time when it is already unbearable. In 1980, when a comprehensive major medical deductible was $50, a 10% increase in premium might have been $180 per year. If you accept an average individual adult cost of medical care at $10,000 in 2019 (admittedly a very arbitrary figure) that same 10% increase is another $1,000 out of the family budget.

I intend to address three primary supply side components of the US healthcare cost structure:

- The facilities component
- The provider component
- The R_x component

RATIONAL CHOICE AND DEMAND

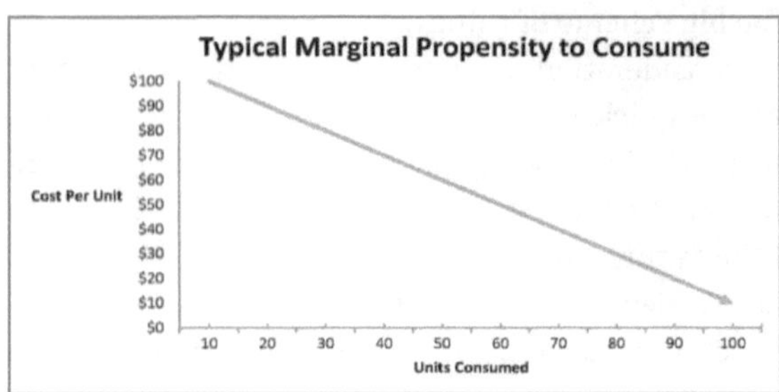

Figure 1

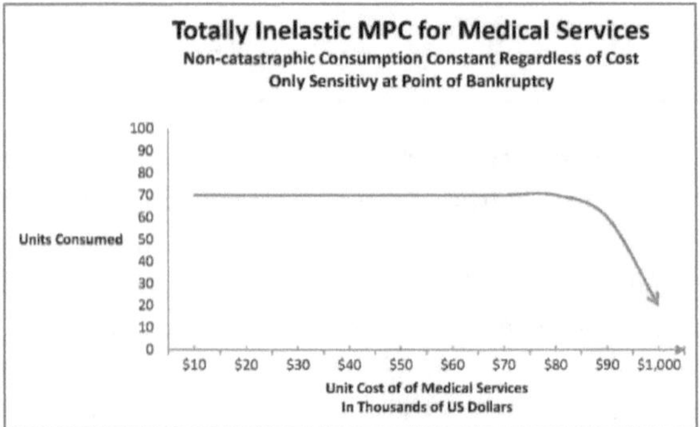

Figure 2

It would be too easy to point the finger at those who provide the vast plethora of services in the US healthcare system and call them gougers. In fact, in most cases they are merely capitalists doing what capitalist do; albeit, there are a few nice people inadvertently doing bad things as well. The hard fact is that the US healthcare delivery system is a totally bastardized economic model. In fact, I am actually sorely tempted to use a more descriptive expletive.

Any business student who has ever taken an intro economics course learns about the equilibrium point between supply and demand. There is an absolute assumption that underpins it; both consumers and producers must be rational in their decisions regarding scarce resources. In that model, they are sensitive to production costs, market pricing and available margins. Economic decisions are made on those factors. In the US healthcare delivery system that is not the case.

Lack of rational choice is the reason. It is an absolute fallacy that patients make price-based choices on the most expensive procedures (*n.b.*, 80% of total costs). In reality, they do whatever they are told by their physicians. Big deductibles and other cost-sharing mechanisms increase the pain; however, they rarely change aggregate demand behavior.

Economists refer to it as the coefficient of elasticity. In the healthcare system, the developers, manufacturers and distributors of cutting edge goods and services know that they can charge virtually anything they want and demand will not change (*i.e.*, within a range bounded by the inanely ridiculous at one end and alternative sourcing at the other). It's referred to as perfect inelasticity. The US abets that process with patent and import protections which effectively guarantees sole source pricing.

Those are the obvious economic choices that professional businesspeople make to maximize profits. I call it the "jug curve" because at the very high-end of potential pricing, there is actually a diminishing point of consumption. At moderate pricing levels, that doesn't exist. The trade-off between units sold and margin per unit is optimized somewhere in the jug – at that point gross revenue is equal for both.

In cases where non-professional boards run facilities, the elasticity issue still applies. Philanthropic, community fundraisers often push administrators to build the most attractive and technically advanced units even when the necessary payback utilization might be known to be problematic. Due to inelasticity, the facility can ultimately charge whatever it wants; it's a matter of maintaining a high enough reputation. Nobody will leave town for a less expensive facility; moreover, the attending physician likely has privileges at the local hospital and prefers to use it. Managed care contracting has skewed the relationship a bit. CFOs have become more sensitive to their relative costs structures. However, little old ladies with access to big money still heavily influence things.

CHAPTER III: *THE PUBLIC'S MINDSET*

Ultimately, healthcare policy is a function of *questae ad publica scriptor* – the public's mindset. Without consensus, policy goes nowhere. One political party just lays in wait for an opportunity to slay the other on the issue. Unless there is a grand commonality of thinking, most initiatives will face an incessant battle for survival. However, in the final analysis, it's not wrong-headed people in DC who will forge long-term policy. It will be the American population writ large who send them to Congress with an absolute mandate. As such, Joe Lunchbucket has as much responsibility to address the existential imperative as any person in America. My personal opinion is that he actually has more; his vote and that of his fellow workers will be the most powerful catalyst for change. Due to the impact on himself, his family, his friends and his job, he must send the folks in DC a message that using healthcare as a wedge issue will cause them to be unseated. Indeed, that message was delivered pretty clearly during the last mid-term elections.

It's important to note that the message to which I refer was hardly as dire as the one that has yet to come. For the most part it was based on short-term, personal considerations: elimination of ACA without an explicable alternative; fear of major costs increases; the return of pre-existing exclusions; and, the elimination of premium subsidies. However, even those relatively narrow issues caused a sea change when the Democrats gained a majority in the House of Representatives. It also important to note that many voters who believe in 90% of the GOP agenda voted against its candidates based on its healthcare stance. I don't find it at all incongruous that political ideology was proven to be less important than personal and family welfare.

Nonetheless, with great power comes great responsibility. I could easily make the argument that for any major healthcare initiative to be successful, it will need at least 67% of the electorate behind it – preferably more. It would be much more useful to our own welfare if 80% agreed on the direction. Clearly, if the electorate is split along party lines nothing substantive will ever get done short of heavy handed mandating.

Given the above, every American has choices to make. One thing we should all agree on: the present system is not sustainable. As a diver in Mozambique once said to my CO after inspecting our ship's sonar dome following a grounding, "*Senhor*, she's there but she's very broke." No amount of grandstanding or short-sighted policy making is going to change that fact.

Of course, how you perceive just how broke it is depends on where you sit – in some cases quite literally. If you are a nonagenarian in your last few years of life it may not seem broke at all; those folks plan on checking out before the bovine excrement impacts the air circulator – so to speak. If you are a twenty-five year old couple with a one year old - and another child on the way - the future might appear bleak indeed. If you are a forty-five to fifty-five year old corporate middle manager in relatively good health, the cost increases might be mildly alarming but absorbable. Of course, virtually none of them have spent time analysing the actually dynamics and the policy alternatives. Many of their feelings about healthcare delivery come simply from watching cable news.

That of course brings up the second elephant in the room: politics in general. Americans are not hand-fed facts; they are force-fed hot words with nebulous definitions. I personally have come to hate the world socialism. It's not because I loathe the concept; it's because the word is used as a cudgel to scare people. The demagogues draw a straight line between anything associated with it and un-American, anti-capitalist thinking. George Orwell wrote about Nineteen Eighty-Four and was an ardent democratic socialist. Today, cable news non-reporters would likely call him a pinko communist rather than a world renowned author.

My point here is not to convince people of one political viewpoint or another. I simply state the above to indicate that the concept at-hand is complex and that there are those in our government who are not above misleading people to gain their own ideological preferences. When one hears phrases like Medicare-for-all will strip you of your right to choose your care; that universal healthcare means there will only be one plan design; that single payer means all insurance companies will go away; or, that socialized medicine is akin to communism, it is important to note that someone out there is probably trying to sway opinions by appealing to latent fears that many Americans harbor.

If the stakes were no more than whether pre-existing exclusions should remain or whether the risk pool should be enlarged by mandating, it would be one thing. Unfortunately, that is not the case. I reiterate again, it is not a discretionary choice any longer; action – correct long-term action - is an existential imperative to protect our maturing generations.

A CASE STUDY – HRAS IN 2019

There are those in DC and elsewhere who would prefer Americans take their eyes off the ball; if they flash a shiny bauble perhaps that might be possible. This week a new initiative was proffered in DC. It is an enhancement of the Health Reimbursement Account mechanism. In this iteration, it would allow employers to provide pre-tax money to employees to purchase individual health insurance policies. I won't even attempt to discuss the impact on employer sponsored health plans or the lack of requirements for essential coverages. Those are important considerations but only tangential to my discussion here. The more important consideration is the psychological impact on people.

All throughout this book I call them stair step initiatives – one-off shots at cost control. In this case, employees – and employers too if they want to terminate a group plan – are asked to watch the shiny new concept while the costs continue to roar out of control behind it. By rolling out an innovative initiative, it makes it appear that the government is really doing something about the actual proximate cause of the oncoming tragedy; don't be dissuaded - they are not. Nonetheless, perceived concerns by the US ratchet down that twenty-five year old couple's fear factor a couple of notches.

The truth is much uglier. It is another type of nipping around the edges of the problem short-term while required long-term solutions fail to get debated. Yet, Americans – even as they start to circle the drain – are relatively satisfied with that level of performance from their elected officials. As such, the latter won't stop rolling out shiny objects until they are forced to do so. It's unequivocally up to every American – individually - not to be taken in by such machinations.

NOT IN MY BACK YARD

Sadly, there is another human trait that impacts policy making. I have consulted with many large employers – both in the public and private sectors. I saw the scenario play out more times than I like to remember. The annual claims bill would come in 10-15% above the previous year; the CEO would be calling for blood from his benefits professionals. They would come to me; subsequently, I would offer undeniably sound alternatives to dampen the cost acceleration. Somehow, between my lips and the CEO's ears my recommendations got lost.

One might ask how that could possibly happen. The answer is actually quite simple. In mid-sized companies – let's say between 350 and 500 employees – the benefits team is often a duo made up of the CFO and the Human Resources Manager. In the public sector it is often a solo act – the entity's Risk Manager. Conversely, I sat in meetings several times in Memphis and Miami, respectively, where national companies fielded dozens of benefits staffers. The structure of the benefits decision making team is the answer to the above rhetorical question.

With one particular client, I saw the CFO repeatedly fail to pass along my recommendations to the CEO (company founder and Chairman of the Board). Every alternative I suggested was parsed for the impact it would have on that person individually. Of course, most of the considerations were financial. However, a few were ideological (*e.g.*, refused to anonymously data mine in their claims history for pointers to future large claims due to it having "big brother" implications; vis-à-vis high blood pressure and obesity to stroke potential). Regardless of the underlying causation, many solid recommendations were never implemented due to personal bias – certainly not well-founded financial analysis. The CEO never knew he was being snookered; yet, his perception of me as a consultant reflected his general dissatisfaction with a claims bill that went up significantly every year. Indeed, he thought I wasn't giving good advice to his team.

Why do I include that anecdote here? People might agree on my existential argument. They might even agree on what structural changes in the healthcare delivery system make the most sense over the long-term – at least hypothetically. However, the moment they intrude on a person's strongly held beliefs or perception of personal welfare, all bets are off. It is like, "Yea I know the city badly needs a new sewage treatment plant; however, I'll vote against any plan to build it in my back yard." My opinion is that, if the guys at Normandy had that same level of pure self-interest, nobody would have gotten off the landing craft. To address the healthcare imperative, Americans will absolutely have to look outside themselves and to the welfare of our society in general. It is not as altruistic as it may sound; the return on investment is undeniable. Caring for the welfare of society doesn't mean giving something to someone who hasn't earned it; it means caring for every American regardless of wealth or position. Personally, I would rather have a country made up of 100% healthy people than a country with 25% super-healthy, 25% extremely unhealthy and 50% at the mean. I don't think it would take a Wall Street genius to monetize my proposition. Why is it so damn hard for some to grasp?

THE GREAT MEDICARE EXPERIMENT

The spectre of socialized medicine was first raised in 1965 as Medicare was enacted under Title XVIII of the Social Security Act. As might be expected, the American Medical Association was its most vocal opponent. The legislation was signed into law by a left-leaning Democrat; however, the idea had been nursed along by prior Republican administrations which saw the need in the post-war era. The doc's anger notwithstanding, it was truly a bi-partisan effort to get it across the finish line. However, in retrospect, President Johnson was the real deal-maker-in-chief (*i.e.*, unlike other pretenders to the title). His expertise at knowing where to squeeze the legislature was legendary. Conversely, he knew where to bend. In addition, as a Texas Democrat, party was somewhat of a relative term for him. Most importantly, he had been elected as the Senate Majority Leader eleven years earlier and knew where most of the bodies were buried around the Capitol.

Today, fifty-four years later, almost 20% of all Americans are covered by some form of Medicare (Parts A through D). Add to that 9 million veterans in the VA system and another 9.4 million in the military retiree TRICARE system. Add two more layers: employer and government managed care organisation plans. Medicaid is provided to roughly 25 million beneficiaries via HMOs and at least 100 million employees utilize some form of employer-sponsored managed care plan. In total, about 66% of Americans get their health care through some kind of regulated system. I am assuming here that the 34% balance is all fee-for-service or uncompensated indigent care. [Note: Some of these numbers could be substantially off stand-alone; however, the concept and conclusions are valid.]

The AMA railed against socialized medicine in '64 and '65. With over 200 million Americans in plans with non-physician controls of one sort or another (*e.g.*, practice protocols, mandatory second opinions, hospital pre-certifications, specialty referrals, Rx formularies, etc.), the same folks would be apoplectic today. However, it clearly proves that substantive structural change in the delivery system is not impossible with the right leadership. Unfortunately, managed care – in whatever flavour – has only dampened the cost structure on a one time basis; it is one of the stair step initiatives whereby a new baseline was established. Although, in fairness, negotiated contracts with all the component parts of the system have caused managed care annual price increases to run below those in the fee-for-service sector. Utilization management savings have actually persisted from year to year; the rates of services don't grow but neither do they generate incremental reductions. Overall, shaving a little off the top hasn't substantially impacted the existential issue; although, it likely slowed its rate of acceleration somewhat. One thing is certain; all the regulated initiatives *in toto* haven't bent the demand curve as a function of component pricing. In fact, I am personally aware of one of the major entities which receives abnormally high pricing on a key consumable due to its lack of flexibility. They haven't bent the curve; instead they have just absurdly pushed the actual price point to the right per Figure 2 above.

CHAPTER IV: *MISSION OBJECTIVES*

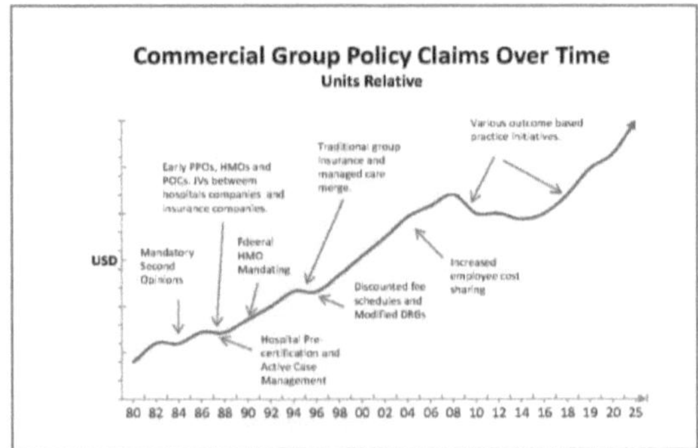

Figure 3

Earlier I mentioned that I was recruited for the First Healthcare War in 1980. Clearly, I meant that to be an amusing allusion – however not entirely. It would require an entirely separate book to do that subject justice. However, I will try to hit a few of the high points here.

I see the war as having had three distinct campaigns. The first began in the early '80s. The second was from the late '80s through the '90s. The third has been the ACA era and its aftermath. Let me call them the Utilization Campaign, the Managed Care Campaign and the Moral Campaign, respectively. I will address the Utilization Campaign first.

THE UTILIZATION CAMPAIGN

When major employers first started to ask health insurers to come up with ways to arrest large annual claim increases (*n.b.*, nominal by today's standards) they responded with new programs. In addition, there was a nascent HMO industry and the first significant PPO was operational. The latter two addressed cost control but were not yet really a market force. All the early innovations were initially directed at wringing waste out of the delivery system - *i.e.*, eliminating what was perceived to be overutilization. The first targets were the docs. Some got incredibly angry when put in the crosshairs; however, their asses were hung out a country mile. Rates of utilization for precisely the same morbidity were all over the map in the US and that fact had become well documented by irrefutable, published studies. They weren't small utilization deviations from the mean that could be explained away by regional standards, population ethnicity or religious proclivities. They were major differences from location to location that appeared inexplicable beyond docs just practicing to whatever their respective markets would bear.

The most efficacious tool in those days was the mandatory second opinion. Initially, it wasn't benefit driven (*e.g.*, 80% if you get one and 50% if you don't); it was all or nothing. As one would expect, the docs who were overturned were mortified; after their appeal to a medical panel was also denied, they were often fit to be tied. One of the ways they fought back was through what I will call here the "coding skirmish." Some docs with time on their hands actually went to classes to learn how to unbundle and rebundle ICD-9 codes to beat the system. Example one: A woman in Florida was in the midst of a nervous breakdown due to family problems. She was admitted for a week to a large city hospital under a "severe dehydration" diagnosis. It was a favour from her doc; he thought he was doing the best thing for his patient. Example two: an OB-GYN in Middle Tennessee couldn't get a discretionary procedure approved. He simply changed the code and threatened the insurance company with a week of inpatient costs versus an outpatient day surgery. He won that battle; insurance companies weren't ready yet to get into the business of forcing practice protocols on docs. It should also be noted that in many small towns throughout America, the local hospital was a willing abettor to such scams. Hospital precertification programs hadn't arrived yet; however, they were on the way.

That leads me to the second phase of the Utilization Campaign – the hospitals. Their asses were hung out almost as far as the docs. On a comparable procedure and morbidity basis (*e.g.*, age, sex and severity adjusted) average inpatient lengths of stay were hugely different from one geographic location to the next – indeed, often hugely different from one side of town to the other. They too were maximizing their censuses by allowing patients to linger longer than medically required. Just like the docs, it was simply a matter of whatever the market would bear.

The insurance companies fought back. On the front-end they demanded that all inpatient hospital stays be preapproved. Diagnoses were checked against histories and planned procedures were checked against diagnoses. A certain number of bed days were then authorized. On the back-end, insurance companies hired nurses to actually make rounds in certain hospitals. It was the advent of active case management and a harbinger of things soon to come with managed care.

Overall, the overutilization that was wrung out of the system in the early '80s never returned. Young docs graduated from medical school in the interim and just accepted the new baseline as the norm. The sting of the external controls never fully went away with the older docs. However, by now, most of them have retired. Example three: I once attended the monthly Board of Directors meeting for a large multi-specialty physicians group in a Florida city. Eight docs were there. Seven of them couldn't have cared less about managed care. Yet, one highly visible old specialist railed on and on about the death of fee-for-service medicine. The other seven didn't necessarily agree with his militarism; however, they followed his lead anyway.

THE MANAGED CARE CAMPAIGN

By the mid '80s the docs were hot as a pistol due to the early cost control innovations. However, they really hadn't seen anything yet. The US had gotten behind the concept of HMOs; if one was granted federal qualification it could force local employers to offer it as an option via "mandating" (*n.b.*, probably the first use of that ugly word relative to the healthcare delivery system.). Most docs and many hospitals considered HMOs an existential threat. To participate in an HMO docs felt that they had to: (1) give up fee concessions (*i.e.*, capitation for primary care and deep discounts for specialty care); (2) agree to a primary to specialty care referral system; and (3) accept patient management oversight by a third party medical director. Initially, the hospitals were expected to: (1) agree to prognoses based lengths of stay; (2) provide access to case managers; and, (3) deeply discount inpatient stays. Later, that morphed into much more sophisticated contracting relationships (*e.g.*, modified DRGs, non-DRG packaged pricing for certain procedures, and dozens of permutations thereof).

I was an active participant in the Managed Care Campaign. In fact, I saw my share of the healthcare combat that was going on in the mid '80s. One of my first assignments was to travel to eight US cities and do feasibility studies for my company. In all but one of those locations we had a nominal HMO presence (*i.e.*, all brick and mortar staff models) via a stand-alone sister company. We were planning a spring offensive. Traditional group health insurance and HMOs were going to merge into what is now called a POS (*i.e.*, Point of Service) plan. I had to examine each city and assess how ready it was for the new concept. I reported back through the traditional part of the company. My bosses really sent me out because they needed eyes and ears in the HMO camp. They didn't fully trust the renegades.

One of the cities I visited was in the Midwest. My company didn't have an HMO there yet; however, it was a key market and an acquisition was being contemplated. One of my objectives on that trip was to secure a fee schedule that was being maintained by a non-profit, collegial organization. To get around price fixing liability, it was always cited as a "maximum allowable" schedule; docs could charge less if they wanted to do so – none did. My company wanted to use it as a baseline for other pricing decisions as it expanded its presence in that city. I had a contact there whose brother was a doc. I asked him if he could get his hands on the fee schedule. I was taken aback when I found that docs in that city considered it a top secret document; albeit, culpability was everywhere on the price fixing. As such, the collegial organization to which I referred above had sworn them all to secrecy and non-proliferation. Eventually I did secure it; however, the handoff to me was right out of a spy thriller.

I also was involved in hospital skirmishes in Florida. In all three cases, I – along with a couple of colleagues – was summarily directed to leave the premises. Each time we had approached the administrator professionally and with deference. However, the person with whom we were dealing felt like they were holding aces. One of those was in Miami. It is my strong opinion that in the mid '80s collusion and price fixing were rampant there. All the docs and hospitals were putting up a united front against managed care expansion. The companies eventually got around the senior doc stonewalling by picking off young ones who needed incremental patients in their growing practices. That was always the spiel; agree to the MCO's rules and pricing and they would get more bodies. It actually worked for many years; however, once every doc in town joined every MCO in town, patient shifting became impossible. However, by that point it also wasn't necessary; the new paradigm was well-established.

The hospitals proved to be a harder nut to crack. In fact, while being walked to the door of one of the three hospitals that ejected me, the chief of staff had the temerity to tell me that our next meeting should be cancelled; he had called his counterpart at a competing hospital down the road and secured a non-cooperation agreement from him as well. He had effectively closed 25-35% of the market to my company with his personal intransigence and one telephone call.

As an aside, the other two hospitals that tossed me were in South and North Central Florida, respectively. Incongruously, not a single one of the three was owned by a for-profit hospital company. It was a matter of lax Board of Trustees oversight in all three cases. The little old ladies to whom I referred earlier were being hoodwinked by administrators who had their own personal agendas. Although in their defense, it was unusual in the '80s for an administrator to last more than two or three years at a hospital. When the admitting docs told them to jump, they were expected to do so.

THE MORAL CAMPAIGN

With managed care well ensconced in the healthcare delivery structure, people took their eyes off the ball. The cost component was still out of control and the elasticity curve had not been bent substantively. However, there were other legitimate battles to be fought in the First Healthcare War as well. One of the most pressing was the 40 million Americans without formalized healthcare protection. I have already mentioned the pragmatic aspects of not allowing such a big percentage of the US population to languish. However, I really think the folks who got behind ACA in 2009-2010 did so more out of moral conviction than anything else. In essence: it's just damn wrong to have all those people bare while others are well-covered (*e.g.*, the federal employees plan). I won't get into the healthcare as a right versus earned privilege argument. However, I feel strongly that the sole purpose of government is to maximize the welfare of all its citizens – not just some of them. As such, we should probably be looking for the best compromise for the entire population. One might think of it as a kind of best fit regression line - not perfect but the best for the entire data set as a whole.

The Moral Campaign is likely to be a protracted one. There will be more skirmishes where short-sighted people attempt to disenfranchise fellow Americans. ACA will be attacked at the margins for years to come. However, short of absolute political suicide, I don't see the elimination of ACA happening. What I can foresee, is folding it into one of the new initiatives I suggested above.

Frankly, I don't believe the anti-ACA camp has the chops to come up with an interim alternative – let alone a long-term solution.

WHO ARE THE BAD GUYS

I am actually not sure there are really many. The original claims cost problem just kind of gravitated to a critical mass. The supply and demand issues are the result of an open market economic system and human idiosyncrasies. The original recalcitrant docs were just trying to preserve a way of life. Hospital administrators and their board members only attempt to maximize community resources.

Possibly the people up in the Midwest with their super-secret fee schedule might tend to the more evil side. The chief of staff who colluded with his buddy would fall into that category as well. The CFO that cost her company money because she didn't personally agree with certain options wasn't totally clean. The DC pols who attempt to tear down ACA for purely political gain should also have to spend some time in the penalty box. Executives who accelerate amortization at the expense of the public also have some questions to answer. However, none of those people have acted out of purely nefarious intent. Nevertheless, I have seen a pretty good approximation of it.

In the early 2000s I was asked to be a panellist for a discussion regarding the future of healthcare. It was held in Boston and it was sponsored by well-known international investment bank. There were dozens of analysts present from various funds. In addition, executives from every major company in the sector made a presentation. I remember one CFO quite specifically. During his presentation, he bragged quite brazenly about cooking his books. It was unlikely as he described it – he would have had to be under audit scrutiny by his CPA firm. Nevertheless, it was his attitude that bothered me. He was quite content with screwing the system – his sole motivation was his bonus. I also had lunch with three young, Big Pharma, microbiology research guys. They weren't planning on gouging the system short-term; however, their motivation was equally unnerving. As I listened to them, I realized that none of them were in the business for altruistic reasons. To a person, it was their intent to discover the next blockbuster drug and get rich - if human kind was enriched along the way then so much the better.

There are also those who attempt to disrupt healthcare initiatives for other reasons. I once worked with a national firm which was in the process of installing a state-of-the-art managed care option for its non-bargaining employees. The company was struggling and the concept would have saved it millions of dollars going forward. In addition, the insurance company involved agreed to waive $6 million already owed to it for two reasons: (1) they doubted it was ever going to be recoverable; and, (2) a leasing arrangement made it the largest de facto creditor. The only way to keep the lease payments coming was to make sure the company didn't go belly up; the cost of the items the leases were on had been expensed years earlier.

Even though it was truly a dire time in the company's history (*n.b.*, they were acquired during a bankruptcy proceeding six months later), their primary union's leadership decided to make an attempt at derailing the managed care initiative – even though not one of their members was to be effected. It seemed to me like a pre-emptive foray relative to the next bargaining round (something which never occurred). It was a national union and quite influential in many ways. Senior management was cowed by the local and regional presidents. They both showed up at meetings to which they weren't invited and asked questions designed to make the initiative seem anti-employee. The insurance company was 95% non-union and they made sure to tell every employee that it couldn't be trusted. The essence of their message was that management was screwing the little guy again.

I can say quite unequivocally that I would put those two on the evil side of the ledger. In an effort to accomplish their objectives, they killed a company and put thousands out of work.

✷ ✷ ✷

Given my experiences in the First Healthcare War, I think that it would be naïve to believe that bending the curve will be much easier than what took place in any of the three campaigns. It could likely – actually will probably – get nasty. That is the pain of all major structural change in a democracy. I personally think we will be measured by how we deal with it.

CHAPTER V: *THE COST COMPONENTS*

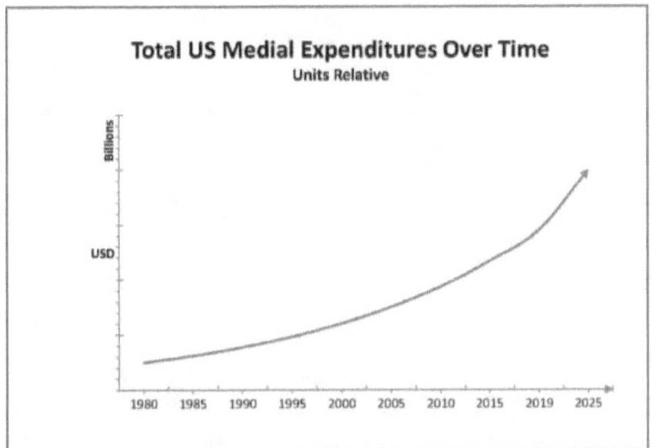

Figure4

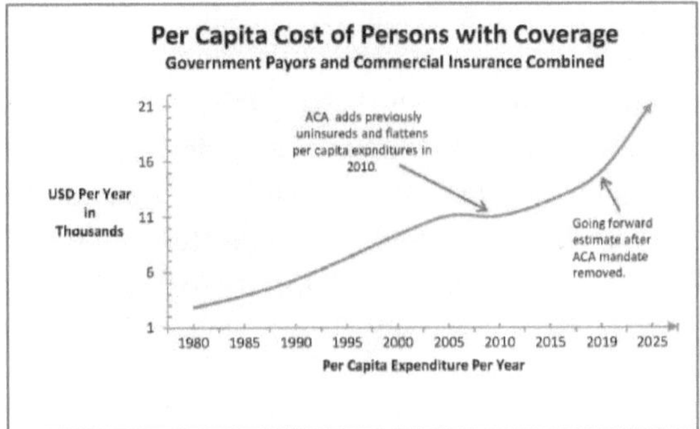

Figure 5

Virtually every effort to control healthcare costs to date has addressed either unit cost or the rate of utilization of services. For the most part they have been efforts to externally force elasticity into the demand curve by making it price sensitive. However, it is important to note that all the efforts to date have been directed at the retail level. The results of managed care notwithstanding, the results have been pretty dismal; in fact, it has been like spitting into the wind. Small shifts in discretionary utilization and moderate pricing pressure (*i.e.*, via negotiated fees and rates) haven't come close to offsetting annual increases in the primary wholesale cost factors.

Beneficiaries have seen their out-of-pocket costs go up substantially every year (*i.e.*, as a percent of all healthcare dollars expended). In addition, physicians and hospitals have seen their gross margins squeezed by the MCOs. That, in turn, has put a little elasticity pressure on the wholesale demand curve – but just a little. For the most part, costs at the wholesale level have abated very little – if at all. It has just been a matter of who has paid for the annual increment. Purchasing behavior – that is to say, perfect inelasticity – has hardly changed at all. It's primarily due to what I call NPS - negligent pass-through syndrome.

Facilities are best positioned to ignore wholesale cost increases. For arguments sake, let's say they can pass along 90% of a 25% wholesale increase (*i.e.*, in the aggregate). If the local MCOs have no viable alternative to that facility, they have to accept the 22.5% increase in cost as a new baseline. They might absorb a small part of the pass-through via reduced product margins (*e.g.*, 10% of the 22.5%); however, ultimately the balance (*e.g.*, 90% of the 22.5% or 20.25%) will go into their retail pricing structures. Unfortunately, the ultimate user of services has nowhere to pass it; they are the ones stuck with it. If you accept that facilities make up half the total medical cost of any program, the out-of-pocket hit at the retail level would be roughly 10% of the total medical cost – or perhaps 8.5% of total premium. And that's just one line of service.

At every level there is a floor pricing below which no facility will go. The MCOs can pound on them during multiple rounds of negotiation; they won't budge – nor should they. Wholesale costs are not in their control; although, for-profit hospital chains, hospital management companies, and hospital purchasing cooperatives have pooled enough purchasing power to, in some cases, effect relative wholesale pricing. However, for the most part, that is only a cost shift; it simply means some other facility is paying more.

Docs are a little less prone to NPS. It wasn't always the case. Terms such as "usual and customary" or "usual and prevailing" were once used to describe how the vast majority of their pricing was established. All acceptable pricing levels were a function of recent historical trends; as such, there was lots of room for abuse (*e.g.*, the de facto price fixing in the Midwest that I mentioned above). All instances of a certain procedure; in a specific geographic area; during the same period of time were arrayed highest to lowest by cost. A line was drawn where 80-90% (*n.b.*, percentiles varied from company to company) of the instances fell below it. That was the new accepted maximum for that procedure; anything above it was considered an outlier from the norm in that area. The concept is still around; however, with 60% or so of care coming through regulated entities, negotiated fee schedules based on some form of RVS (*i.e.*, relative value scale) are much more prevalent. In addition, much primary care is done on a capitated basis (*i.e.*, a flat fee per assigned patient each month whether seen or not) which makes it impossible to know how an individual procedure is compensated. Although based on certain assumptions, capitation levels can sometimes be reverse engineered.

If only 40% of procedures are now on a fee-for-service basis, the percentile method is statistically questionable. To increase the size of the data set, larger geographical areas are required for analysis; that dampens local idiosyncrasies and induces localized error. I think it actually might end up being a double edged sword. It seems to me that the percentile levels and the negotiated levels are being drawn towards one another. If they merge, MCOs will no longer have any physician costs advantage over other forms of delivery; albeit, they will still have the most utilization control.

***

I've almost ignored the utilization side of cost control. As I mentioned in prior chapters, to date the initiatives have been virtually all stair stepped. A one time, lower baseline utilization was established; however, wholesale percentage cost increases didn't abate at all. The result of each effort was that initial savings from a reduction in utilization was offset quickly by cost increases for the utilization that remained. In essence, the rate per thousand population for a given procedure might have been structurally lowered permanently; however, total costs for those procedures in the same population might be higher than the starting point within a few years. Albeit, it can be argued that the annual increase in absolute dollars was permanently reduced as well; a percentage increase was applied to a recurring smaller number of procedures.

FACILITIES

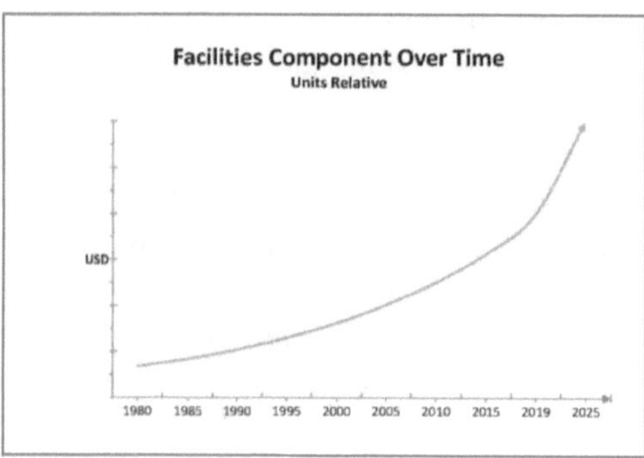

Figure 6

By facility I mean primarily acute care hospitals. Though, certain other kinds of brick and mortar entities could be grouped with them as well. What I don't mean is assisted living facilities, on-premises skilled nursing hybrids, nursing homes, and the like. Many of those have similar cost drivers but they tend not to have inelastic demand. In addition, I don't consider them to be an existential threat to the US. Albeit, the concept of thousands of 90 and 100 year old Americans drifting around bankrupt and without a place to live in the year 2119 could certainly be the basis for another book.

Figure 6 above is based on "relative units" because the actual dollar amounts are meaningless to my argument. The most important thing is the slope of the curve. Please note three things: (1) the trend has been significantly up for over forty years; (2) it has been continuous regardless of external utilization and pricing pressures; and, (3) the slope of the curve has gotten more acute in recent years.

Second opinions, utilization management, managed care, and more efficient physician practice paradigms haven't slowed unit cost acceleration at most hospitals. I ascribe that primarily to the NPS I mentioned above. They might have reduced America's total hospital bill in the aggregate. However, cost per unit of service is still a runaway freight train.

I think for-profit hospital companies have huge potential in terms of bending the curve. They have the strongest reason to push back on suppliers; their officers have a fiduciary responsibility to maximize shareholder value. They are well positioned to combat arbitrary pricing. So why don't they? If you are an administrator of one of those facilities you want to do two things: (1) minimize through corporate leverage your wholesale costs; and, (2) slide your retail pricing in just slightly below the best not-for-profit hospital in town. That sweet spot renders the highest gross margin. However, the latter shadow pricing of the competition doesn't result in an aggregate reduction in costs. It merely shifts purchasing advantage to corporate profit margins. The slope of the curve does not flatten.

How can facilities bend the curve? Is it actually possible to change purchasing behavior of individuals based on pricing? Will a person buy one less bed day based on a lower rate? Of course, the likely answer is that hospitals don't have that kind of clout. However, just like a manufacturer of a healthcare product, they do have control over their cost structures (*e.g.*, capital investment in new units, etc.) and how much they pass along via NPS. While Americans are weaned away from the concept of buying a healthcare good or service at any cost it is offered – perfect inelasticity – hospitals should strive for long-term price competitiveness.

I feel strongly that ultimately all hospitals will need to get there. That's actually the essence of bending the curve (*i.e.*, priced based purchasing behavior and market efficiency). They might as well start right now. In addition, corporate and community healthcare leaders should step up as a vanguard; nothing will happen in DC without broad professional support. Indicating that they see the absolute inevitability on the horizon – and the dire consequences of inaction – would give the matter the underpinning it needs.

PROVIDERS

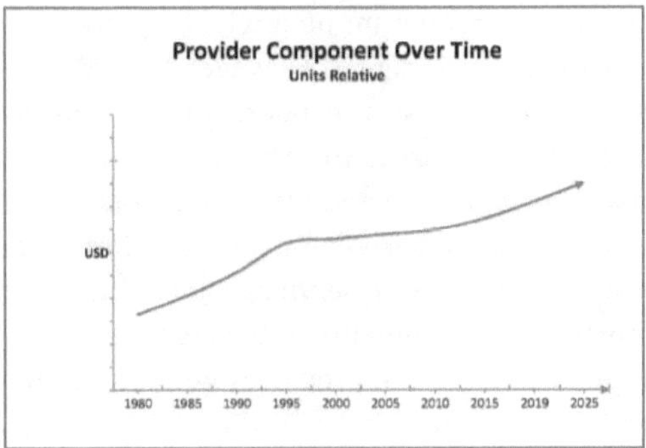

Figure 7

By providers I mean physicians. As I described in detail earlier, from second opinions to managed care, the docs have been pretty well beaten up during the last forty years. They have seen pricing pressure and third party practice oversight.

Both induced significant depression on the older generation of providers. As I said earlier, most of those folks are now retired. The new generation of docs take this environment as a given. Essentially, it is the one into which they were born. They have also been given new marching orders. The post-dinner speaker one night in the JFK School of Government dining room spoke to the docs about their futures. He told them point blank that, between PA-Cs and the Internet, all the low hanging fruit was going to be picked off. For them to remain relevant as clinicians, they would have to concentrate on the 20% of their practice that required their higher level training and expertise. The subliminal message was that 80% of what they did could be done by non-docs. It was a hard message to deliver; however, the young docs weren't totally surprised by it.

I see very little pressure to return to the excesses of the early '80s. Although, I think the fee-for-service Medicare utilization rates are absurdly high due to there being virtually no oversight. The occasional horror stories of fraud that come out of retirement areas like Miami or Tampa are actually only a drop in the bucket compared to the legal looting of the system. However, there is some good news too.

Figure 7(Provider Component Over Time) shows the slope of provider costs over time. Like the facilities costs in Figure 6(Facilities Component Over Time), the actual cost units are meaningless. The slope is the indicator to watch here too; overall, it is pretty flat. I personally think it reflects the dampening of physician pricing by managed care. In the '80s the slope was still pretty steep. However, as a higher percentage of procedures came through MCOs, it tapered off after about '95. It is reasonable to see an annual increase in fees comparable with a change in the consumer price index; as such the constant upward slope is predictable.

I am quite sure that docs will be forced to cost shift quite dramatically in the near future. I don't see the total amount of services nor their unit pricing going up (*i.e.*, beyond the historical average). However, if Medicare and Medicaid reimbursements are reduced across the board due to politics or the threat of system bankruptcy, docs will be forced to recover the lost revenue elsewhere (*n.b.*, the same could actually be said if wasted utilization was wrung out of Medicare). Any entity that has a fee schedule based on a percent of Medicare payable could be similarly affected. Given that 60% of services come through a contracted entity and that a sizeable portion of the remaining 40% is fee-for-service Medicare (*i.e.*, under a fixed schedule) where are the providers going to go for it? The answer is: likely no place. I don't foresee the balance of the system being able to sustain the required subsidy. I do see two results: (1) the curve in Figure 7 gets flattened a bit temporarily; and, (2) all hell breaks loose in the world of docs. As with the facility leadership, this would be a good time for the physician leadership to step up as the vanguard of a new paradigm. One thing is certain; the US will never return to the good old days of the '80s and '90s. Bending the curve will be inevitable and one-way only; in addition, it will be one hell of a tough slog. The best and brightest I met at Harvard should be commissioned as frontline generals.

Can providers bend the curve? The answer is yes - perhaps more than any other part of the delivery system. Americans need to be weaned from the "any price goes" mentality. As I said at the top, in many ways Americans are healthcare junkies; for the most part, it's a psychological addiction. Docs can assist their patients – and the system as a whole – by inducing pricing versus utilization sensitivity. For instance: buying a CABG (*i.e.*, coronary artery by-pass graft) package for $100,000 in Atlanta or the exact same package for $25,000 in Jacksonville; alternatively the patient might be counselled on an option to forego the procedure completely and be tracked annually while on meds. A really forward looking doc might even mention a couple of offshore sites; a few have training and outcomes at least as good as those of the US. Of course, all those options require moral courage.

Indeed, discouraging business at the local heart mill might make a doc a pariah. I actually saw a form of that in Ft. Lauderdale in the early '90s. A large group of nationally renowned cardiologists had moved into town and set up shop. Long-established cardiologists effectively embargoed them by forcing hospitals to withhold the granting of admitting privileges. The new docs had deep pockets; they just went to the well and purchased their own hospital – a little rehab job that was priced to sell. Once it was clear to the other local hospitals that the new guys weren't going away, they immediately granted privileges. However, it was too late; a big chunk of the cardio business had gone down the street.

I heard a story from an Executive Director in a mid-sized southern city. He and a doc - who was to become Medical Director - were sent there to build a brick and mortar staff model HMO. The market was binary around two major local hospital systems (*n.b.*, both not-for-profit). Another national MCO had set up a staff model a year earlier and used one of the two systems exclusively. When they came into town, they attempted to set up a relationship with the other system and its staff docs; however, the overture was summarily rebuffed. They returned to their home office and reported the mission as a failure. Nonetheless, it was another case of deep pockets. The city was a market in which their company wanted to be. They were sent back - essentially with a suitcase full of cash. They built a good sized clinic and recruited docs from all over the US. They then threatened to sue both hospital systems for privileges. Along the way they became federally qualified and mandated every major employer in the county. It was obvious to the hospital system it wanted to use that they weren't going away either. It granted privileges to all the new docs. Just like in Ft. Lauderdale, a huge amount of market share was already lost by the long-standing docs who tried to initially embargo them. I heard that the new HMO had been prepared to bus patients over a hundred miles away to a hospital with which their parent company had a contract. However, the hospital administration and its staff docs blinked first.

PRESCRIPTION DRUGS

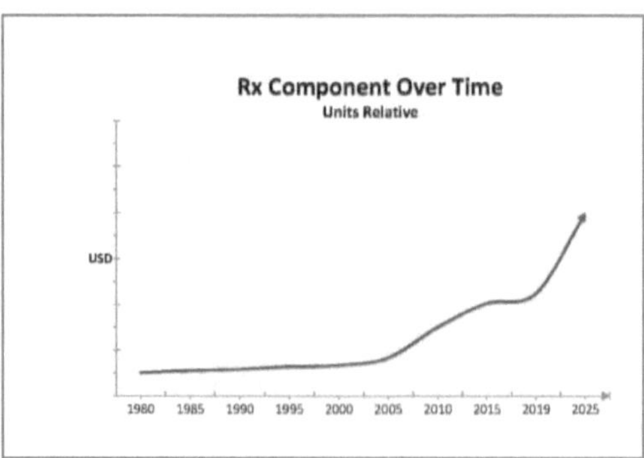

Figure 8

Prescription drug costs are one of the least controlled parts of the healthcare delivery system. R_x costs have had a general upslope since 1980 but in the last 10–12 years they have accelerated dramatically. The cost driver is primarily wholesale pricing of brand drugs. However, abetting that process is a patent system that is gamed to keep generic equivalents off the market. To the extent that manufacturers can keep a drug "sole source" they can charge ludicrous prices for it. If a brand name drug is the most clinically efficacious – that is to say the docs really have no alternative but to prescribe it – the manufacturer can charge any price they want. Once again, it is a case of perfect inelasticity. Price will not alter the purchasing behavior.

Timing is also an issue. With managed care pressure to avoid surgical procedures wherever possible, prescription drug regimens have become systemically more important. In fact, I predict that utilization per capita for R_x will only continue to rise (*i.e.*, in units prescribed).

Big Pharma makes the argument that American R&D allows for the development of "blockbuster" drugs every year. As such, they roll out exotic drugs to treat highly complex, low incidence diagnoses. It posits that to recover the R&D investment the industry must charge extremely high prices for drugs that are sold in very limited quantities. However, they fail to mention a few points.

I already mentioned the goodwill amortization issue. It's front–end loaded and charged primarily to US consumers. The exact same drug might be sold overseas for a fraction of US pricing. In a perfect world, all the R&D investment would be spread over the pricing of all the drugs in the system – brand and generics alike – and the offshore pricing disparity would be mitigated (*n.b.*, based on purchasing ability versus the moral imperative of certain drugs being available, some skewing is justified). Once equitably spread, amortization schedules would have to be extended out. There would be no sensible argument for front-end loads (*i.e.*, other than cash flow and corporate profitability). R&D would not necessarily have to take a hit in terms of absolute dollars allocated to it; though, more debt might just have to be carried on balance sheets and reduced earnings due to interest charges accepted.

The US might also want to consider shifting a higher percentage of prescribed drugs to an over-the-counter status. It's not that the system cannot adapt to such. The issue is really how to ensure more open access isn't abused. There are myriad ways to make that happen. Indeed, many drugs that require a prescription in the US are already OTC in other countries. I had personal experience with such when I caught a dose of the crud while in Mexico. I was able to go to the local *farmacia* and get what I needed without ever seeing a doc. That same drug requires a prescription in the US (*n.b.*, along with a primary care visit copay to get it).

There have been attempts to bend the R_x demand curve via formularies and multi-tiered pricing systems. One who wants the latest and greatest brand name drug pays the most for it. If there is a generic equivalent, and the person is willing to use it, he or she pays the least. The formulary might require generic-only for a group of well-established drugs. When there is more than one source for essentially the same therapeutic value, formularies normally adopt the least expensive. Of course, formularies and multiple tiers are only used in regulated systems. Pure fee-for-service has no such limits.

Docs tend to prescribe generics when they are forced to by formulary or when it is a well-established drug (*e.g.*, a common blood pressure drug or NSAI pain killer). However, they are reluctant to order anything other than brand names when the therapeutic equivalency is a bit blurry. Moreover, at times they have no option. When the diagnosis is complex or rare, brand drugs - still under patent - might be the only prudent way to practice.

* * *

Above, I gave both providers and facilities a moral pass in how the US got to the present state of perfect inelasticity. In many ways they were components of a delivery system that just drifted into that state with very little nefarious intent. Unfortunately, I can't give Big Pharma that same indulgence. In its case, I feel strongly that corporate greed is the dominant factor. It isn't reacting to forces that it only marginally controls. Indeed, the industry operates quite independently of most of them. A new, sole-source (*i.e.*, under patent brand name), blockbuster rollout can be priced as far right on the demand curve as a pharmaceutical manufacturer wants; short of an alternative, docs will prescribe it and patients will buy it at all price points.

* * *

Bending the R_x demand curve won't be easy. It seems to me that it is beyond the capabilities of MCOs, providers or facilities. To bend the curve, a certain drug would have to be arrayed by price. Subsequently, a doc would theoretically have to write a script with financial bounds (as directed by the patient based on choice of price point). Docs would also have to be trained to prescribe on a price versus marginal efficacy basis. For instance: at what price point should less of a certain drug be prescribed - or a different, less expensive one considered? Is the marginal clinical value equal to or greater than the marginal cost?

To get a complete formulary arrayed by price is a virtual impossibility in the current system. Patents and import restrictions simply won't allow it. Many drugs on any formulary that might be established would still be arbitrarily priced (*i.e.*, to the extent it is not a supply and demand related decision).

Changing physician prescribing behavior will be just as hard. However, certain financial inducements could be offered whereby they would assist patients with price sensitive purchasing.

Perhaps, alternatively, third party service bureaus might even be established whereby an analysis could be done on behalf of the patient and the doc sign off on a chosen course of action prior to the R_x purchase. The doc could stick to medicine and the service bureau could do all the heavy analytical work.

* * *

To address the existential healthcare imperative, my personal opinion is that the regulation of Big Pharma has to go through a drastic structural overhaul. The issues with the industry are profoundly entrenched – almost bunker bomb proof *à la* the National Rifle Association. In addition, the fixes required to bend the curve are complex on a myriad number of levels. Various US laws would have to be changed to affect the desired outcome – from accounting to competition. An entirely new set of interrelationships would have to be developed. Nonetheless, it seems to me that our representatives in DC cannot continue to protect a single segment of the healthcare delivery system at the expense of the welfare of all Americans over the long-term. It might be painful to Big Pharma executives; however, it will hardly be more so than it was for docs and hospitals during the earlier campaigns of the First Healthcare War. The difference in this case is that the battles won't be led by large employers and insurance companies. It is imperative that they be led by the US government on behalf of all its people.

CHAPTER VI: *TARGET MARKET BEHAVIOR*

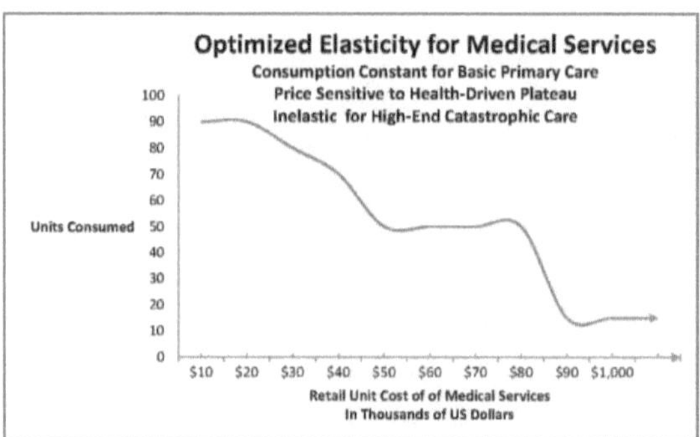

Figure 9

Consider Figure 9 above to be the end result after bending the curve I initially showed in Figure 2 (*i.e.*, the straight line, perfectly inelastic curve). Once again, the units are relative. It simply shows how the number of units consumed drop significantly as the price increases. One can look at it as an individual healthcare item or the entire system as a whole.

I have assumed the far left end of the curve to be primary care level pricing. Over a narrow range, the consumption doesn't change. However, above some arbitrary price point that behavior changes. As costs increase, consumption goes down, as per a typical demand curve (*e.g.*, Figure 1 above).

Ultimately, there is a plateau; consider it a minimum number of units that <u>must</u> be consumed on a non-discretionary basis. A fairly broad range of pricing exists for those goods and services over which units consumed stay constant – regardless of price.

Moving further right on the curve, I have assumed dramatically more expensive – but relatively discretionary - goods and services. Once again, units consumed lessen as costs increase.

The very far right of the curve shows it going back to perfect inelasticity. It reflects human willingness to pay virtually anything to stay alive when faced with a catastrophic diagnosis. It probably should show some downward slope; neither an individual nor the system as a whole has unlimited resources.

***

I freely admit that Figure 9 is no more than informed speculation on my part. However, the relationships are reasonable – even if not scientifically founded. The numbers of units produced and consumed are likely less that at present. Unit pricing also reflects significant demand sensitivity at various price points. As such, rollouts and annual increases are effectively bounded.

Indeed, if the assumptions hold true, then the curve would have been successfully bent and an American healthcare imperative effectively addressed. The essence of the challenge to get there is strictly in the courageous execution of innovative policies. Like that diver in Mozambique reported to my ship's CO, "*Senhor,* she's there but she's very broke." As such, this is no time for the fainthearted to point toward halfway measures.

#

APPENDIX A: *GRAPHS*

A.1: TYPICAL ELASTICITY CURVE

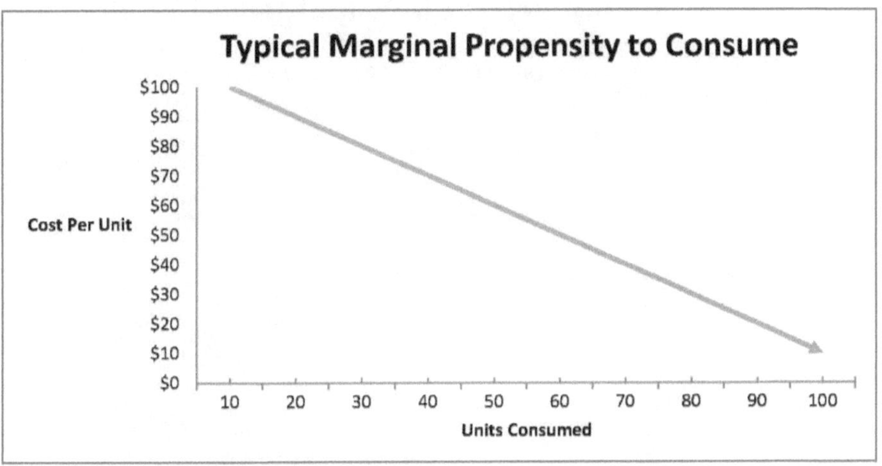

A.2: ACTUAL INELASTIC CURVE

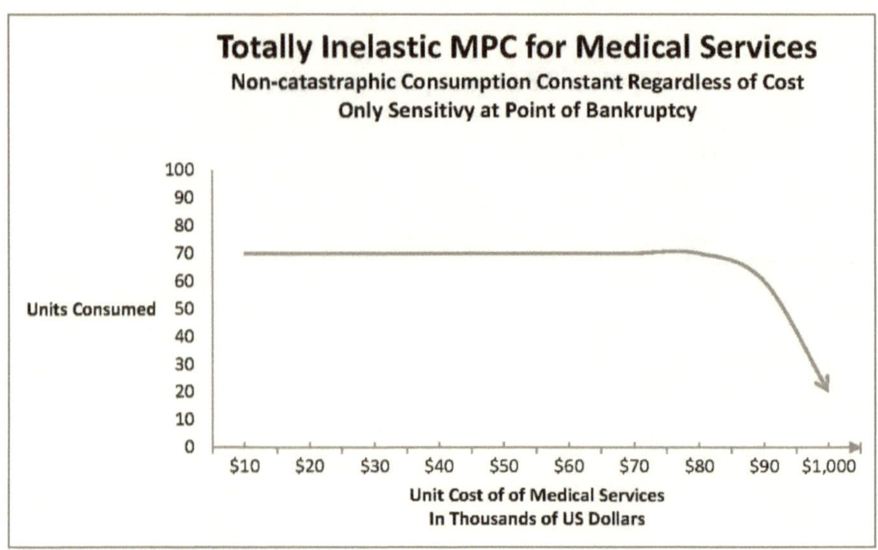

A.3: TARGET ELASTICITY CURVE

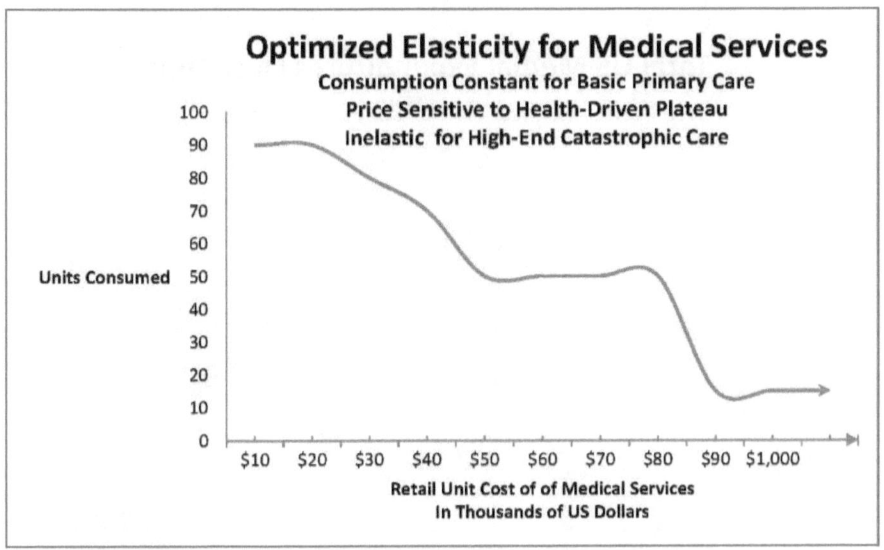

A.4: TOTAL COST OVER TIME

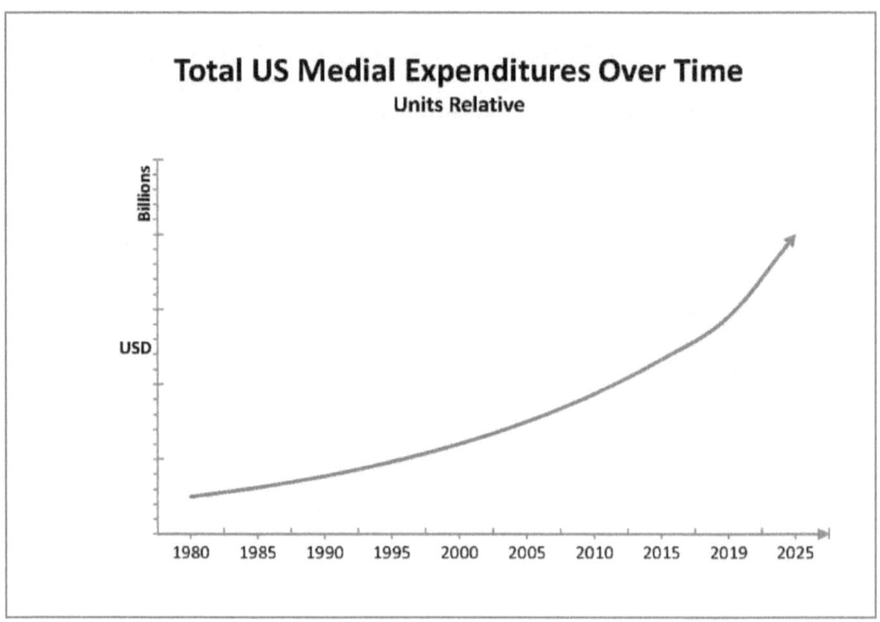

A.5: COMMERCIAL INSURANCE CLAIMS

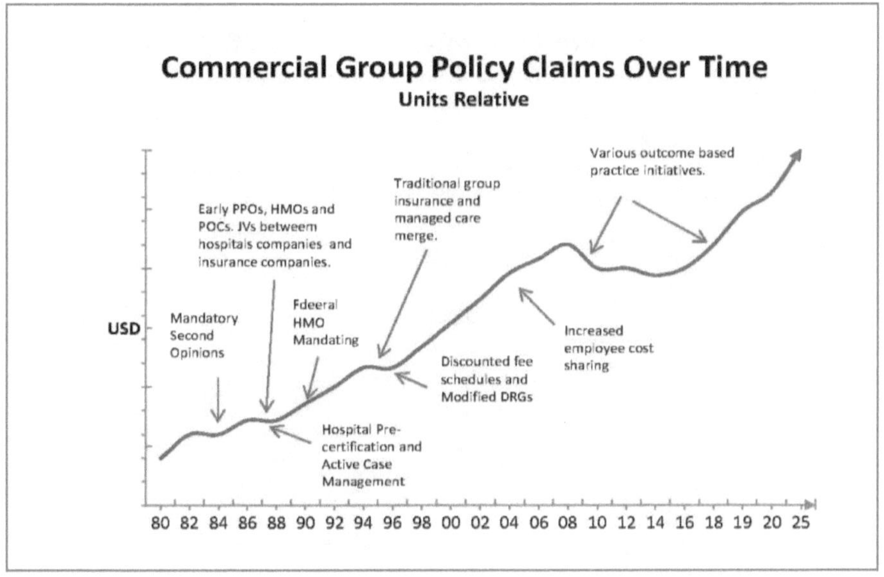

A.6: PER CAPITA COST

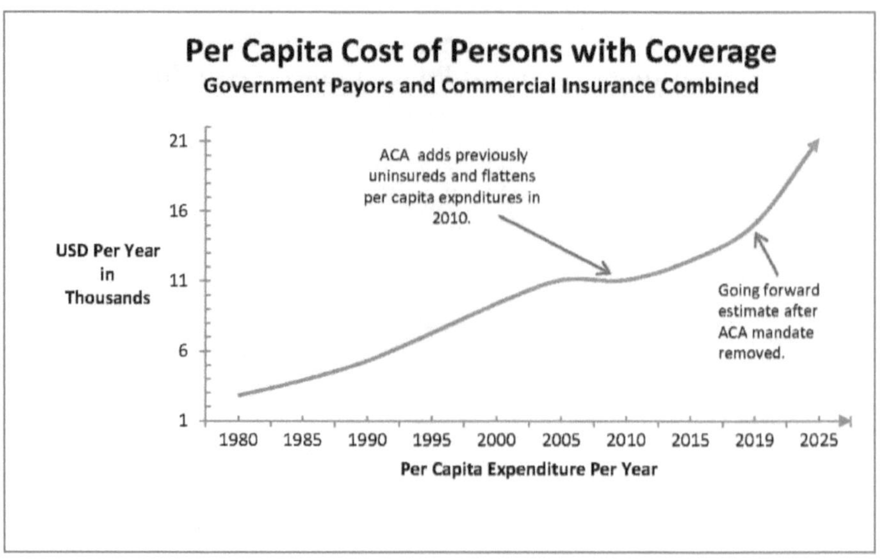

A.7: FACILITIES COMPONENT COST

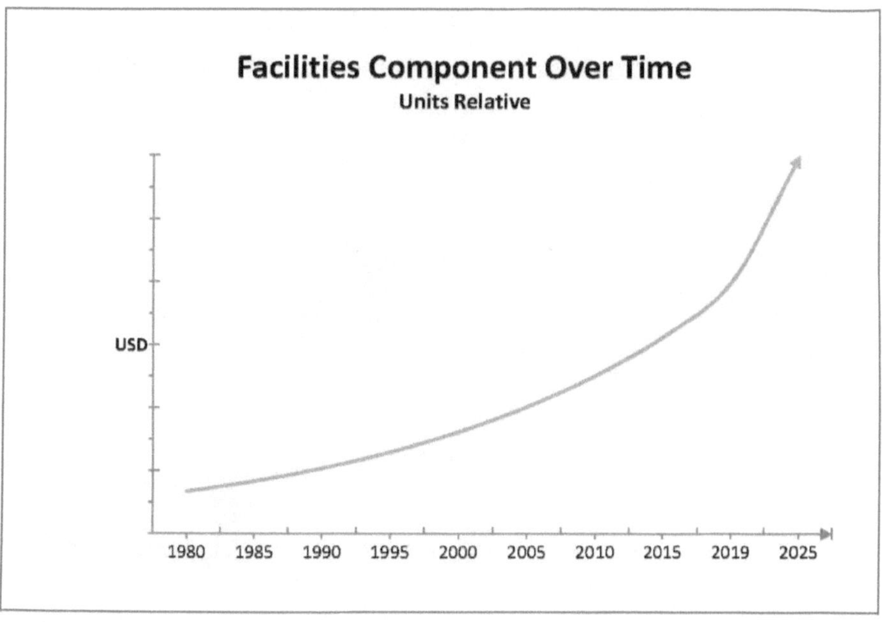

A.8: PROVIDER COST COMPONENT

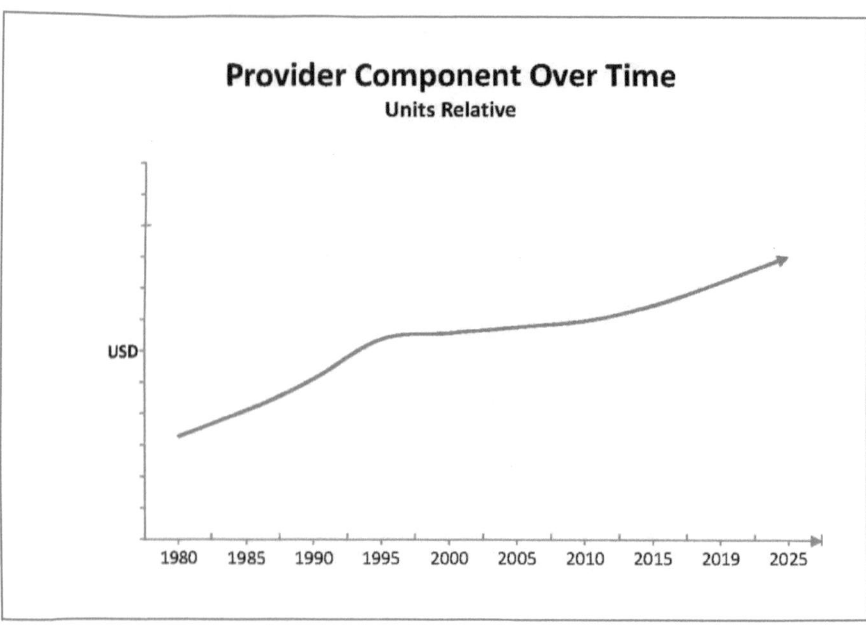

A.9: RX COST COMPONENT

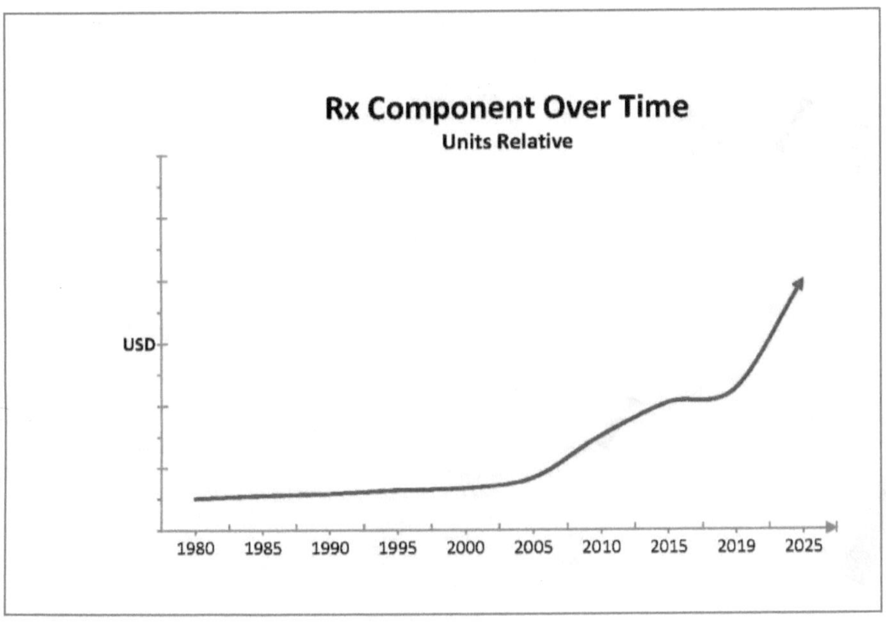

APPENDIX B: MISCELLANEOUS

B.1: HARVARD CERTIFICATE

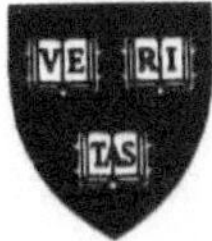

**HARVARD MEDICAL SCHOOL
HARVARD SCHOOL OF PUBLIC HEALTH
JOHN F. KENNEDY SCHOOL OF GOVERNMENT
HARVARD DIVISION OF HEALTH POLICY RESEARCH AND EDUCATION**

This Is To Certify That

Robert W. Murphy, MBA, REBC

was enrolled in the executive Program in Health Care Policy entitled

Skills for the New World of Health Care
March 7 – 12, 2004

*Harvard Medical School is accredited by the Accreditation Council for Continuing
Medical Education (ACCME) to sponsor continuing medical education for physicians.*

*Harvard Medical School designates this educational activity for up to 41.5 hours
in category 1 credit towards the AMA Physician's Recognition Award.
Each physician should claim only those hours of credit that he/she actually spent
in the educational activity.*

_______________________   3/12/04   _______________________
Faculty Chair   Date   Faculty Chair

____
Faculty Dean for Continuing Education

This Page Left Blank

www.ingramcontent.com/pod-product-compliance
Lightning Source LLC
Chambersburg PA
CBHW032130050726
47590CB00008B/3024